I0119078

Presented
To:

_____

By:

_____

On:

_____

Scripture taken from the HOLY BIBLE, NEW INTERNATIONAL VERSION®.
Copyright © 1973, 1978, 1984 by International Bible Society. Used by permission of
Zondervan Publishing House. All rights reserved.
The "NIV" and "New International Version" trademarks are registered in the United States
Patent and Trademark Office by International Bible Society. Use of either trademark requires the permission of International Bible Society.

Living Without in Peace
Workbook
Asantee Asche' E-Faye Mitchell
Email: aae.author@gmail.com
www.ourgoldenmic.com

ISBN: 978-0-578-87473-9
Publishing Company: Efaye Inks LLC

No part of this book may be reproduced or transmitted in any form or by any means, electronic or mechanical – including photocopying, recording, or by any information storage and retrieval system—without permission in writing from the publisher. Please direct your inquiries to aae.author@gmail.com

Table of Contents

Dear friend,

I am proud of you for getting this book. This shows you are ready to take the next steps in grieving properly and/or help someone along the way of grieving properly. This book educates you on matters you may or may not have gone through. It will also educate you on realizing what is happening with your loved ones. I had the privilege of interviewing Kaylah Mitchell; she is my sister who walked along side me through one of the hardest moments of my life. Throughout this book, you will see the manuscript of the interview. Her insight will shine light of what grieving can look like from another perspective.

Before you delve into this book, understand that this will be painful. Healing and growing can stretch you in ways that may be uncomfortable. Notify someone that you are reading this book and encourage them to read it with you. This journey is a journey you should not do on your own. Telling someone close to you will help because you will go through emotions that you have tried to hold in, having an accountability partner when you have episodes will help you stay grounded in the process.

I want you to know that I am walking this walk with you. Although I am not there physically, I am visible through the words on these pages. Understand you will get through all things with the help of Jesus.

Dedication

I dedicate this book to anyone that has lost something in their lives. Loss is a difficult thing to process, and life is even harder learning how to live without. This book is to let you know you are not alone in this walk of emptiness you may feel. Losing a family member, a friend, a pet, or even an opportunity is tragic and is unexpected. We must fight through it and take it one day at a time. You may not have experienced this pain, but you may know someone who is going through it. Nonetheless, this is still a great book for you. Not only can you both do this together, but you sure can help them along the way. Educate yourself on this matter. We are here to give hope that brighter days are ahead. There is no guarantee that the feelings may go away, but we can learn to manage them. We want to educate you on every stage of grief while the author gives her personal experience with them.

Thank you for choosing us to guide you through this journey.

About the Author

I am no doctor, therapist, nor psychologist. I do not have the authority to diagnose or prescribe medications. These tools I give you come from years of creating a formula that helps me deal with losses in my life. These tools have helped me and the ones around me Live Without in peace. I am here to share my findings with you. I have attended numerous grief and loss classes and sought therapy. I encourage you to do the same. This book will assist you with the day-to-day work you will need when your heart feels heavy. I am a Professional Life Coach and I have helped clients work through numerous trials of life - grief being one of them. I know how difficult it can be to experience a great loss. I am almost a decade in, and I still feel pain, however, without the support around me, I would not be here helping you.

Thank You

Thank you to everyone who displayed patience toward me during each stage. Thank you for the professionals that created the grief and loss classes.

Tykeyria Green, thank you for coming to rescue me from my thoughts with listening and speaking my love language with quality time.

Khalilah Mitchell, thank you for kidnapping me and taking me to the beach when I had episodes. Allowing me to breathe and release the frustration I had from the moments that felt unbearable.

Mommy (Victoria Mitchell) Thank you for answering your phone every time I called. Thank you for loving me when I did not know how to love myself in the mist of the storm. Thank you for providing the help I needed even when I did not believe I needed it. Thank you for placing the right people in my life, at the right time for each stage of my grieving.

Kaylah Mitchell, last but most definitely not least. I appreciate you for walking this walk called life with me, through the great and devasting times. Thank you for rocking with me even when the boat tipped over. My grief caused you and Mom grief, right now I pray my healing brings you both healing. I love you.

Definition

Without- in the absence of.

Peace- freedom from disturbance; tranquility.

It Sucks...

It sucks when your dog runs away and does not come
back.
It sucks when you did not come in first place in your track
race.
It sucks when a friend moves away.
It sucks when you lose a scholarship.
It sucks when you did not get accepted into the college you
wanted.
It sucks when you lose a job.
It sucks when you lose a spouse.
It sucks when you lose a pet.
It sucks when you lose a family member.
It sucks when a relationship ends.
It sucks when you lose yourself.
All are considered a loss and you may grieve in different
ways.

~Asantee Mitchell

Living Without in Peace...

What are you living Without?

_____

_____

_____

_____

_____

_____

_____

_____

_____

***Being Without*-** I am living without my brother.

***My Loss*-** I met my older brother when I was 15 going on 16. My mother found him on Facebook. I was not cool with my father's side of the family at the time. So, she found him, and my brother connected me to my entire paternal side. We got very close over the course of 2 years. We spoke about any and everything. We experienced a love that neither one of us have experienced. From a long-lost brother and sister to newfound twins. We tried to make up for lost time and it was the best time of my life. I did not know too much about my fathers' side at the time, but my mom wanted everyone to come together for my Sweet 16 party. To picture this moment, my birthday was a family reunion with my mothers' side, my father's side, and my adopted side all under one roof. Even though my brother could not make it, we still celebrated my moment together. In my senior year of high school, I found out he left me. He was in a motorcycle accident and died. Because I was still in school, I was not able to go to Trinidad for his funeral. I honestly do not think I would have been ready to go. I lost my best friend, whom I had for only two years. However, I am so glad I had two years with him, compared to none.

For the purpose of this book, I had to go back and do some research. During that time, I found a conversation between us that made me cry and die laughing in the same minute. We were supposed to celebrate my 18th birthday together, and we would be inseparable when we visited each other. He told me about every one of my family members and to this day, he was accurate about all of them. He prepared me as much as he could. Living without my brother peacefully took years. I am now to the point where the thought of it will not shut me down and ruin my day to now being able to tell my story. I can share moments of him with laughter and a bright smile on my face.

Living without in Peace. Living in Peace without my brother looks like when Facebook sends reminders of us, I sit in admiration instead of anger. I am reminded of how much he loved me instead of being without his love. That older brother's love is something different. No one is like him. No love is like his love.

5 Stages of grieving.

1. Denial- you tell yourself it is not true. You cannot accept the fact that you are now without. This looks like disbelief and downplaying possible consequences of the issue.

My Denial- The day my Brother passed away, my mom had my sister take my phone to make sure I did not get on social media or talk to anyone until she got home. She had to be the one to tell me. I am glad she did what she did. I thought my mom was playing when she told me my big brother was gone. The first thing I did was laugh like I just spoke to him. Then I cried all night, telling God this cannot be true. I thought about calling him just to make sure he was actually gone.

Interview with Kaylah

Asantee- What did my denial look like to you?

Kaylah- You talked about your brother as if he were

still with us currently, even after you knew he passed. You

would talk about the conversation you had with him as if

you just had them. Nobody could say anything about him,

talk about him, or mention his name. You listened to all his

songs, every day! No radio, or Beyonce whom you love.

You just consumed yourself with everything of him. You

did not want to hear he was gone, and you would tell

yourself he was just sleeping.

***How to Get Through Denial*-** Honestly examine what your

fear is. Acknowledge the facts of what has

happened. Allow yourself to express your fears and

emotions in a safe way like writing, dancing, or

hiking. Think about the potential negative consequences of

not acting. What are you blocking yourself from and who are you blocking out?

2. Anger- This can look like being mad at the world. Fragile, snapping on everyone and at any chance. Possibly being destructive, mentally, physically, and emotionally to yourself and or others.

My Anger- To this day my sister would tell me things that I have done, and I do not recall them. Nine times out of ten, you are taking anger out on the ones closest to you that do not deserve it. I went through a period of rage and I would black out often. I would go off on my sister a lot...I went off on teachers just for looking at me wrong. I was ready to fight anybody at any time. I blamed God and was so upset with Him for taking my only Big Brother from me.

Interview with Kaylah

Asantee- What did my anger look like to you?

Kaylah- Your anger was so sporadic. I feel like your anger ran into denial; it was almost like you did not completely get out of the denial stage before anger came. You will be talking about him like he still here, everything is okay and then boom. You would say, this is why I do not talk to God, we were just fine, we were doing okay, he was healthy and now he is gone. It was a downward spiral from there. That is when you became rebellious and started doing things you wanted to do even if it was against the house rules.

How to Get Through the Anger Stage- Think before you speak, eat healthy, exercise, meditate or even get massages. Discover what arouses feelings of tranquility for you and invite it into your daily routine. Allow yourself to take time out during the day, giving yourself maybe a 5-minute mental break at work or school just to gather yourself. Seek help if your ways are not helping you, anger management class or even therapy are all get avenues to try.

3. Bargaining- Defense, making a deal. I remember one of the Tyler Perry (as Madea) movies, the son pleads with God saying, "If you give my mom back from her battle of cancer then I would stay off the streets."

My Bargaining- I did not experience this being that I was young and really did not know what this was even though I was angry for a very long time. This looks like pleading. "I'll do this if you do this for me, I'll do right if I get one more chance."

Interview with Kaylah

Asantee- Why do you believe I went through a bargaining stage?

Kaylah- Your bargaining was more so overcompensating, you started acting and reaching out for any attention. Your pleading was not crying to God about change my situation, it was more so, I am throwing away all my morals and at this point you were being ruthless. To me that is pleading. You were asking for help; you need that attention that a child would need to be held. Instead of asking for it, you just broke all the rules. You had the attitude of I am going to do everything I usually do not do because the life I lived before was with my brother. Now I do not have my brother, I do not know who I am, the things I did before reminds me of him. That is bargaining, that is pleading, is it not? You were pleading for help! Your bargaining was extreme, and you did not know what you were going through to reach out for help. You show it in different ways.

How to Get Through the Bargaining Stage- Understand

that this is normal. Join a local support group, talk to a

therapist, family, or even friends. Seeking professional help

is always a great step in the right direction to healing.

4. Depression- This could look like wanting to be alone,

always in the dark, always tired, not doing what you love to

do.

My Depression- I cried a lot and I stayed in my room just

as much. My doctor at the time wanted me to go on

medication that my mother feared would potentially

become addictive. So, a few years later, I went to a family

doctor who recommended natural herbs that I used for two

years. My weight was up and down. I did not want to go

anywhere; my room was always a mess when I was about

to have an episode. I was always tired, I would go to work,

school, and back to my room. I caught depression a little

late from when it started but was able to get it under control. Today, I have been completely healed from depression. Although I get sad, I am no longer depressed. With a lot of Jesus, unwavering faith, and trust, God has healed me.

Interview with Kaylah

Asantee- What did my depression look like to you?

Kaylah- It almost seemed like you just woke up one day so down, you started giving things away that mattered to you. You started saying goodbye dramatically to everybody. A whole speech like I cannot wait to see you guys again, I just love y'all. And we would just be like girl I will see you tomorrow at school, what are you talking about? You always wanted to be outside with your friends but when you got home you were in your room, in bed, underneath the covers. I would ask what is wrong with you and you would always say, I am just tired, I have a lot of schoolwork to do, or I do not feel like cleaning my room. It was so settle that Mom and I did not pick up on it. It was not bad until you started giving everything away. You were such a big drawer, such an artist and loved all your work. You used to sell them and wanted no one to touch it. Those very things you started given

away. Your vocabulary started changing from present tense to past tense. That is when we knew something was wrong.

How to Get Through Depression- When you are having an episode, step away and take a minute to breathe. Acknowledge that you are not okay and breathe through it. Call a friend or family to help you ease the moment to be able to get through the day. Surround yourself with loved ones. Get some sun, take a walk. Feed your body, mind, and soul with healthy positivity.

5. Acceptance- Acknowledging you now must be without, realizing you will never have that thing again. Ready to take the next steps of living without. Being able to breathe. Have more good days than bad!

My Acceptance- I was able to breathe a little bit. I would tell myself, "Bro Bro is not here anymore." In all, I was glad I had that Big Brother's love for the couple of years that I cherished. I am so thankful that the last things we said to each other were, "I Love You." I am glad we knew how we felt about each other and how much we enjoyed each other. That we did not leave this world not knowing our connection and purpose in each other's life. I was thankful to experience such a love. I accept the fact that I cannot call him, and I will never see him in the Earthly realm again. I will never forget the memories we shared. I could tell a story about him and cry out of laughter instead of pain.

Interview with Kaylah

Asantee- What did my acceptance look like to you?

Kaylah- I knew you accepted it in a healthy way, when it was one of his birthdays and you were at work and just received a promotion. Facebook reminded you of your brother saying something like, I love you or something along those lines as if it just happened. Instead of you crying in pain you cried of joy saying to yourself, he is so proud of all my accomplishments. You had a brother sister moment, and it was beautiful to watch. All I could say was, wow, she is doing great with this day. She has fully accepted he is not here but instead of looking at it as a loss, you saw it as I will always have that connection with him. You began to talk about him in a celebratory aspect.

How to Get Through the Acceptance Stage- Understand there are many phases to acceptance but each one is a step closer to living without in peace. Remember to be kind to yourself and the ones around you. Celebrate your

achievements. Every obstacle you overcome is a reason to

celebrate. Spread the word, give someone hope that

they too can get through it.

Each stage may be longer than others. My Denial

took days, but my anger went on for a few years. My

acceptance stage had multiple phases. First, I was accepting

he was gone. Then, I will never hear from him again. To

now able to talk about it. Kaylah's insight to what it looks

like from another point of view is valuable. To hear about

me from someone who walked it with me is an entirely

different level of acceptance I did not know I needed until

writing it down for you. Accepting that healing can be so

ugly but so refreshing.

Different Types of Grieving

Anticipatory Grief- Grieving before your loss. If you find a loved one has an illness and see them declining. Loss of what you would hope for and the realization that things will change forever.

Normal Grief- Any response. Silence, anger, eating less or excessively, tears, loss of interest in hobbies or common practices.

Delayed Grief- Does not affect you until a later time. May become emotional but not fully grieving.

Complicated Grief- normal grieving escalates to long grieving. Stagnates the ability to function at your full capacity. Violent outbursts, suicidal thoughts, guilt, radical lifestyle changes.

Disenfranchised Grief- not associating the loss with reality.

Chronic Grief- denial, feelings of hopelessness or defeat, disbelief. Clinical depression, self-harming thoughts, substance abuse.

Cumulative Grief- back-to-back losses within a short period of time. Does not allow time to properly grieve.

Masked or Inhibited Grief- Unresponsiveness to the emotion, does not show outwardly, private.

Distorted Grief- extreme feelings of guilt and anger associated with hostile, self-destructive behaviors.

Exaggerated Grief- intense normal grief responses. Increasingly gets worse over time. Self-harm, suicidal thoughts, drug abuse, abnormal fears, night moves, often manifest into psychiatric disorders.

Secondary Losses in Grief- primary loss can affect other areas of your life.

Abbreviated Grief- short-lived response to a loss. Commonly having something or someone filling the void.

Absent Grief- does not acknowledge and shows no signs, shock.

Let Us Work!

Identify-

1. What are you living Without?

2. What stage do you feel right now?

3. Do you know you will not get it/them back?

4. Are you pleading?

5. Did you stop doing your favorite things?

6. Are you ready for the next steps living

Without?

_____

_____

_____

_____

_____

_____

_____

_____

_____

_____

_____

_____

_____

My response-

1. I am living without my brother.

2. I believe I am at the acceptance phase with moments of anger.

3. Not as bad as I was, and I feel like I can work through my emotions.

4. No. I am not pleading.

5. I picked up doing a few things I love but covid stopped a lot of things so trying to find new ways of moving,

6. I am ready for the next steps.

Solution/Goal

How would you know you are in a good place without?

_____

_____

_____

_____

_____

_____

_____

_____

_____

_____

_____

_____

_____

My Response- I know I am in a good place without when I do not cry on his birthday and to say his name and think of the good times rather than the painful part where I am without. I know I am there when I could smile while I say his name and blissfully reminisce.

Disclaimer- Understand that it is not terrible to cry on the day, or to the song, or at the place that reminds you of life without. Allow yourself to feel every emotion and to express every stage. Just try not to stay there too long! And be mindful of the ones around you. There were times I was not, and it caused damage.

If you are feeling ___, try -

Anger- Workout, go boxing, take a jog

Sad- Cry just do not cry all day, try to change your crying

into crying for joy.

Happy- Dance with the feeling.

Alone- Want to be alone? Fine, but in the midst; write,

sing, dance, draw, or do something that comes effortlessly

that will allow you to healthily express yourself and what

you are feeling.

Depressed- Want to sleep all day? That is fine as well, it is

okay to rest for as long as your body needs. But you should

always try to get up and get active to make the most of your

24 hours of the day.

Step-By-Step

1. Changing your perspective

2. Making it a goal to get through the day.

3. Allowing yourself to cry.

4. No Time Frame

5. Celebrate

1. Change your perspective- view your loss from a different point of view. Every negative thought, think of two positives.

How will you change your perspective?

_____

_____

_____

_____

_____

_____

_____

_____

_____

My Past Thought Process- I am lost without my brother, I will never experience a Big Brother love ever again.

Changed Thinking Process- I am honored I got to spend the time I did with him. I rather have a couple of years to never have it at all.

2. Daily Goals - make a decision to live without in peace.

a. Wake up, look at yourself in the mirror, and tell yourself it is going to be a good day.

b. Smile! Just move your face, work those muscles.

c. Do not be too quick to react! Listen and then speak.

d. Everyone is going to make you angry, remember, do not react negatively.

e. Understand you are not at your best today, but you are getting better every day. Make it a priority to write out your goals.

What will your daily goals be?

_____

_____

_____

_____

_____

_____

_____

_____

_____

My Goals-

a. Laugh 3 times today.

b. Cry for 4 minutes, not 5 minutes.

c. For every negative thing I think of, I think of two positives.

3. Cry- express your thoughts and feelings.

If you need to step away and cry, do it. At work, tell someone you are going to the bathroom, allow yourself the time you need. Typically, 3-8 mins. Then take deep breaths, clean your face, do a little shimmy, and go back to work. DO NOT HOLD IT IN. You owe yourself that release.

How do you feel after crying?

_____

_____

_____

_____

_____

_____

Me- Cry a river. I used to cry all night almost every day and woke up with my face swollen. To reduce puffy eyes, you can put a cold compress on them. Old cucumbers or a wet tea bag that was refrigerated for 20 minutes helps significantly.

4. No Time Frame- Overnight change is not realistic. It could take months or years to be at a comfortable place living at peace Without. If you see improvement every day, then that is a win!

What are some things you improved in?

_____

_____

_____

_____

_____

Me- I lived without my brother for 9 years now and I still miss him daily. Just this year, I felt like his birthday was more of a celebration than one of the worst days ever.

5. Celebrate- progression takes time.

If you went a day without crying (without holding it in) or not crying of pain but laughter, then go celebrate with ice cream. If you acknowledged you are Without, then have a dance party. If you thought of two positives to outweigh the negative, treat yourself. Reward the success of mental training.

What is the first thing you think of when it comes to a celebration?

_____

_____

_____

_____

_____

_____

_____

_____

_____

_____

Me- I would celebrate a lot with pizza, but I was getting fat

as a result. I had to switch it up and I did a lot of shimmies.

I would call my mom to celebrate and have a movie night.

Say to Others

What to say and Do If You Know Someone Who Is Going
Through Without.

Listen...

Listen.

Listen!

Hugging always is nice but ask first before you run to hold
them. Depending on the setting, some people may need to
be able to come back to reality physically after being held.

"I am here for you."

Acknowledge how bad it is.

Reach out while still allowing them to feel and process
their emotions.

Offer your sincerest condolences to them and their family.

Do not tag grieving relatives in photos of the deceased
online without permission.

It felt so traumatizing for me when people would tag me in my brothers' photo open casket at his funeral. That was the last thing I wanted to see of my brother. I did not handle that well, and it was a huge part of why I lost my mind.

Say to Ourselves

What to say to ourselves...

- "This will not happen overnight."

- "Today is a good day!!"

- Acknowledge how you feel. "I feel.." or "This made me feel..."

- "I made it another day"

- Remind yourself of one good memory.

- "I will not avoid objects, people, or places that remind me of that lost person or thing."

- "I will take help when it is offered. It is going to help me."

- "I will do what I love again!"

How Do I Live in Peace

Without?

- I told myself he is no longer in pain and the two years I existed with him were the best two years of my life.

- We made great memories to tell our siblings when we found each other and my children.

- Focus on the things I can control. I cannot control the fact he is not here, but I can control my thoughts.

- Acknowledge what I am feeling and not ignore it, remembering not to stay there too long. For example, grieving for over 24 hours is not healthy. (set your come back limit)

- Eating Healthy- Certain foods can be too heavy and make you feel low on energy.

- Exercising- It is good for your mental, emotional, and physical health.

- Meditation- Centers and ground you.

- Exploration- Gives the sense of excitement and thrill!

- Being Gentle with Yourself- We can sometimes be the hardest person to ourselves, be gentle like a butterfly landing on a flower.

- Loving Others- Because God loved his children!

- Self-Care- No one can take care of you better than you!

- Seeking Guidance if Needed- Speak to a life coach or therapist if you need to, they help in ways you could not even imagine.

- Forgiving Yourself- It is okay to make mistakes, you are human! Do not beat yourself up.

- Forgiving Others- Forgive even when you do not get an apology.

- Listening to Yourself- Pay attention to your gut feelings and your intuition!

- Speaking Your Love Language to Yourself- Learn your love language and love on yourself.

- Being Content with Saying No- You do not have to force yourself to go or do anything you do not want to do.

- Disconnecting Periodically- Taking a break from social media brings mental health, and a break for yourself gives that peace of disconnect from the chaotic world.

- Living in the Moment- Tomorrow is not promised, love on your family, smile 50 times a day, laugh until your stomach hurts, and capture all the moments you can possibly catch.

Prayer

Daddy,

Thank You for opening my eyes today, thank You for who You are, thank You for another day, thank You for my friends and family and their patience with me along my journey. My heart is broken living Without. I feel damaged, annoyed, frustrated, but I know who You are. You are Lord of Lord, Kings of Kings, You are my provider, my healer, my way maker. I am not okay right now, and I need You to trade my sorrows for Your joy. I am angry and I need You to trade that with peace and love. I do not want to get out of bed, but I need You to help me sit up and move. I need Your strength to get through these days. I need You to give me patience. Walk with me. Hold me, lift this weight off my heart, mind, and soul in Jesus' name.

Amen.

Write A Letter

Ex: I wrote a letter to my brother.

When I was asked to do this, I thought they were crazy. I could never write a letter to my brother. I was asked a couple of times and then I did it. I wrote it on my phone, and I cried the entire time while thinking, "This is real, I cannot hit send and get a response back from him." Then it became a lot easier afterward. When I wanted to talk to him, I was able to.

This practice could be completed in so many cool ways. You could write it and then burn it, write it, and put it in a candle float. You could put it in a glass bottle and let the ocean take it away.

- Pet- Write a letter, what would you say to them right now?

- Job- What would you say to that manager?

- Scholarship- What would you say to the person who took it away?

- Family- What would you say to your loved one(s)?

- Let me help you...

- Start it off like this depending on your loss...

  - Dear Ex-Manager

  - Dear My love

  - Dear My pet

  - Dear My opportunity

  - Dear sibling

  - Dear item

  - Dear me

  - Dear my joy

  - Dear my child

_____

_____

_____

_____

_____

_____

_____

_____

_____

_____

_____

_____

_____

_____

_____

_____

_____

_____

_____

Good Job!

Motivational Quotes

"What is there to do when people die, people so dear and rare, but bring them back by remembering." - May Starton

"We are healed of suffering only by experiencing it fully." - Marcel Priest

"Grief is like the ocean; it comes on waves ebbing and flowing. Sometimes the water is calm, and sometimes it is overwhelming. All we can do is learn to swim." - Vicki Harrison

"How lucky I am to have something that makes saying goodbye so hard." - Winnie the Pooh

Scripture's

Psalm 9:9

"The Lord is a refuge for the oppressed, a stronghold in times of trouble."

Psalm 34:18

"The Lord is close to the brokenhearted and saves those who are crushed in spirit."

Psalm 147:3

"He heals the brokenhearted and binds up their wounds."

Philippians 2:20

"I have no one else like him, who will show genuine concern for your welfare."

John 14:27- Peace

"Peace I leave with you; my peace I give you. I do not give to you as the world gives. Do not let your hearts be troubled and do not be afraid."

Matthew 5:4

"Blessed are those who mourn, for they will be comforted."

Romans 5:3-4

"Not only so, but we[a] also glory in our sufferings, because we know that suffering produces perseverance; 4 perseverance, character; and character, hope."

What Are You Grateful For?

_____

_____

_____

_____

_____

_____

_____

_____

My Response - I am grateful for the time I had with my brother. I am thankful for my family and friends who have helped me get through every celebration without him. I am thankful I have a story to tell my unfound siblings once we are united. I am beyond thankful to God for blessing me with an older brother and never leaving my side as I went through my grieving process. I am thankful for you for taking the next steps on living without peace.

Hotline

If you know someone or you are going through a rough

time, please contact the following numbers for assistance.

If it is an emergency, please call 911

Professional Life Coach: by Asantee Mitchell

Website: www.ourgoldenmic.com

National Hopeline Number: 1-800-SUI-CIDE (784-2433)

SAMHSA's National Helpline: 1-800-662-HELP (4357)

Safehorizon Hotline: 1-800-621-HOPE (4673)

Thank you!

You now have the tools to Live in Peace Without!

How do you feel?

I would love to hear your testimonies.

Send an email to aae.author@gmail.com.

Follow IG: @ourgoldenmic

@aae.author

@aae_marketing

@aae.production

Follow FB: @ourgoldenmic

YouTube Channel: OurGoldenMic

Blog Page: ourgoldenmic.com

www.ingramcontent.com/pod-product-compliance
Lightning Source LLC
Chambersburg PA
CBHW052143270326
41930CB00012B/2994

* 9 7 8 0 5 7 8 8 7 4 7 3 9 *